Contents

Preface

"Pray do not mock me: I am a very foolish fond old man,
Fourscore and upward, not an hour more or less;
And, to deal plainly,
I fear I am not in my perfect mind.
Methinks I should know you and know this man;
Yet I am doubtful: for I am mainly ignorant
What place this is, and all the skill I have
Remembers not these garments; nor I know not
Where I did lodge last night. Do not laugh at me;
For, as I am a man, I think this lady
To be my child Cordelia."

King Lear (William Shakespeare)

This booklet was originally written in 1996 to be used as a component of continuous health education activities, with special emphasis on the diagnosis of dementia of the Alzheimer type, the treatment of concomitant disorders and the management of patient and family by primary care practitioners. We are fortunate that cholinergic-enhancing medications such as donepezil have proven safe and useful in a significant number of persons with Alzheimer's disease. Highlights of results from randomized clinical studies and guidelines for drug utilization have been incorporated into this new edition. Many thanks go to Drs Felix Bermejo, Alexander Kurz and the late Luigi Amaducci who have helped as co-editors in the Spanish, German and Italian translations (respectively) of the first edition, and congratulations go to Alzheimer's Disease International for creating hope for so many people.

SG

March 1999

What is Alzheimer's disease?

Operational definition

Alzheimer's disease (AD) is a progressive neurodegenerative disorder with characteristic clinical and pathological features, although with individual variations for age of onset, pattern of cognitive impairment, and rate of decline (Figure 1).

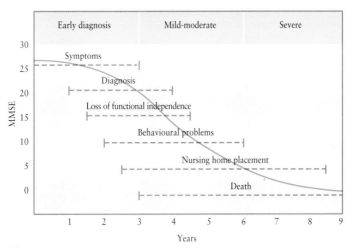

Figure 1
Natural history of Alzheimer's disease (see Feldman and Grundman 1999).

Natural history

AD may be difficult to distinguish from cognitive decline associated with normal brain aging in its earlier stages (Table 1), but the relentless deterioration of memory for recent events, fluency of speech and spatial orientation eventually reduces autonomy for instrumental activities of daily living (ADL) – for example, handling finances. Anxiety and depression may complicate the diagnosis in these early stages, but there is a progressive resolution as insight is lost. In the intermediate stages more and more supervision is required for self-care ADL, and tasks such as dressing and toileting become difficult. In the late stages nursing care in institutional settings is usually necessary.

Stage	Clinical characteristics
1	—
2	Subjective forgetfulness but normal examination
3	Difficulty at work, in speech, when travelling in unfamiliar areas, detectable by family; subtle memory deficit on examination
4	Decreased ability to travel, count, remember current events
5	Needs assistance in choosing clothes; disorientation to time or place; decreased recall of names of grandchildren
6	Needs supervision for eating and toileting, may be incontinent; disoriented to time, place, and possibly to person
7	Severe speech loss; incontinence, and motor stiffness

Table 1
Global deterioration scale (from Reisberg et al 1982).

Symptomatic domains

There are a number of cognitive (Table 2), ADL (Table 3) and neuropsychiatric (Table 4) features of AD, with variable expression in severity of symptoms based on premorbid factors such as education, gender or culture. Unfortunately, we have so far a limited understanding of the neuropathological and neurochemical substrate for most of these symptoms. There is a complex interplay between loss of cognitive abilities, particularly executive functions that have to do with planning, abstraction, attention, and functional autonomy. Neuropsychiatric symptoms are usually the most troublesome for carers.

- Memory
- Language
- Visuospatial function
- Executive function

Table 2
Neuropsychological domains altered in Alzheimer's disease (see Mohr et al 1999).

Instrumental tasks (IADL)	Self-care activities (ADL)
Performance in employment	Choosing proper attire
Handling finances	Bathing
Keeping appointments	Dressing
Handling of correspondence	Grooming
Travelling alone	Toileting
Use of household appliances	
Maintaining hobbies	

Table 3
Loss of functional autonomy in Alzheimer's disease (see Gélinas and Auer 1999).

- Activity disturbances
- Affective disturbances
- Aggressiveness
- Anxieties and phobias
- Diurnal rhythm (sleep) disturbances
- Hallucinatory disturbances
- Paranoid and delusional symptoms

Table 4
Neuropsychiatric symptoms in Alzheimer's disease (see Allen and Burns 1995).

Neuropathology

The neuropathological changes associated with AD have been well described (Table 5), the most characteristic lesions being illustrated in Figure 2. We still have inadequate knowledge of the sequence of events that lead to premature and widespread loss of neurons in this (so far) uniquely human condition. Brain biopsies and autopsy studies have helped shed light on the structural–neurochemical correlations, but an animal model such as transgenic mice would greatly facilitate our understanding of AD (Poirier et al 1999).

- Cortical atrophy
- Synaptic and neuronal loss
- Amyloid angiopathy
- Neuritic plaques with amyloid core
- Neurofibrillary tangles with paired helical filaments
- Acute phase reactants and localized inflammatory reaction

Table 5
Neuropathological changes associated with Alzheimer's disease (see Terry et al 1994).

Figure 2
Characteristic neuropathological features of Alzheimer's disease. (a) Neuritic plaque with central amyloid core (Ag. stain). (b) Neurofibrillary tangles of paired helical filaments (Ag. stain). With thanks to Dr J Richardson, Montreal Neurological Hospital, Canada.

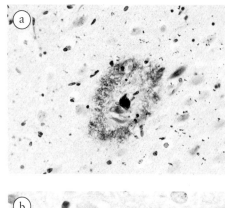

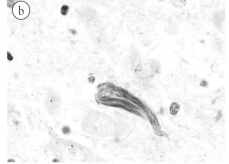

Aetiology

Clues as to the aetiology of AD come from the study of families where AD is inherited from mutations on chromosomes 1, 14 or 21 (Sadovnick and Lovestone 1996). Recent observations suggest that a mutation on chromosome 19 may be responsible for sporadic AD, which could explain up to two-thirds of patients with this condition between the ages of 60 to 80, at least in Caucasian populations (Poirier et al 1993). Patterns of risk and protective factors are emerging from large population epidemiological studies (Table 6).

Protective	Risk
ApoE2 or 3	Age
High education	ApoE4
Use of oestrogens	Family history of dementia
Use of anti-inflammatory drugs	Head trauma
	Low education
	Systolic arterial hypertension
	Down's syndrome

Table 6
Protective and risk factors for Alzheimer's disease from population studies (see CSHA 1994a).

At this point in time, AD seems to be a heterogeneous disorder with an interplay between a number of genetic and acquired factors over a lifetime, converging to a dementia syndrome when a critical number of neurons and their synaptic connections has been lost (Figure 3).

Socioeconomic impact

The prevalence of AD doubles every five years after age 65 with figures in industrialized countries in the order of 4% of population over age 75, 16% over age 85 and 32% over age 90 (Evans et al 1989; CSHA 1994b) (Figure 4). Direct costs are estimated to be in the order of $40,000 per patient, and indirect costs $174,000 per patient, in the USA. Furthermore, they have been shown to increase four-fold as patients progress from mild to severe stages (Hux et al 1998). Delaying the onset of symptoms by five years could reduce prevalence by 50% in one generation. Symptomatic treatments and delaying nursing home placement would reduce costs significantly (Gauthier et al 1999).

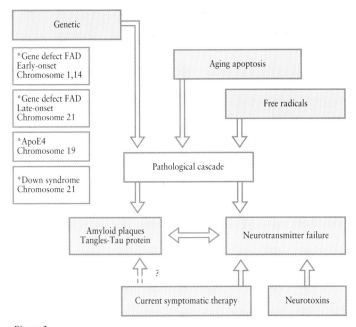

Figure 3
Pathogenesis of the Alzheimer syndrome – a convergence cascade (see Feldman and Grundman 1999).

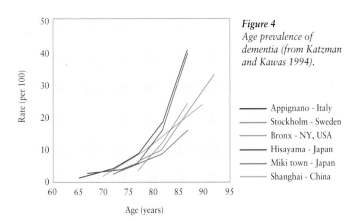

Figure 4
Age prevalence of dementia (from Katzman and Kawas 1994).

— Appignano - Italy
— Stockholm - Sweden
— Bronx - NY, USA
— Hisayama - Japan
— Miki town - Japan
— Shanghai - China

Clinical diagnosis

History and physical examination

It is possible to make a positive diagnosis of AD with knowledge of its clinical features, diagnostic criteria, a good history from a reliable informant and serial observations (Bouchard and Rossor 1999).

The diagnosis of AD requires first the recognition of a dementia syndrome, defined by criteria such as the ones proposed in the DSM-IV (Table 7). As a second step, NINCDS-ADRDA criteria for probable or possible AD are used (Table 8). A reliable informant is essential to the diagnostic process and much more valuable than any laboratory test so far available. Questions must be relevant to cognitive loss, particularly in the realm of memory, language, and orientation. For example, questions about ability to:

- Play card games
- Keep appointments
- Remember names of friends and distant relatives
- Find his or her way in less familiar parts of the city

Multiple cognitive deficits, including memory impairment and at least one of:

Aphasia – Problems with language (receptive and expressive)

Apraxia – Inability to carry out purposeful movements even though there is no motor or sensory impairment

Agnosia – Failure of recognition, especially people

Disturbed executive functioning – Impaired planning, sequential organization and attention

Cognitive deficits severe enough to interfere with occupational and/or social functioning

Cognitive deficits representing a decline from previously higher function

These deficits do not occur exclusively during the course of delirium

Table 7
Modified DSM-IV criteria for dementia syndrome (American Psychiatric Association 1994).

Definite AD	Clinical criteria for probable AD
	Histopathology of AD by biopsy or autopsy
Probable AD	Dementia by history and neuropsychological testing
	Progressive deficits in memory and one other area of cognition
	No disturbance of consciousness
	Onset between ages 40 and 90
	Absence of systemic or other brain disorder causing dementia
Possible AD	Dementia with variations in onset or course
	Presence of systemic or other brain disorder
	Single progressive cognitive deficit

Table 8
NINCDS-ADRDA criteria for Alzheimer's disease (McKhann et al 1984).

The potential impact on daily life of such cognitive changes, depressive elements and behavioural changes must be explored, sometimes with the informant alone if he/she is afraid of embarrassing the patient.

The mental status assessment can be facilitated by the use of standardized clinical tools such as the Mini-Mental State Examination of Folstein et al 1975 (MMSE, appendix 1), but highly educated persons with AD may have normal scores on the MMSE (above 24 points) even in the early stages of AD. Serial observations over time are usually required to confirm a progressive cognitive loss and its impact on instrumental ADL.

The neurological examination is usually normal in AD. Asymmetry of motor signs (tone, speed of movement, deep tendon reflexes, plantar responses) or of release signs (palmomental, grasp) suggest focal lesions of vascular or tumoral origin.

Differential diagnosis

The four 'D's' of geriatric medicine are depression, delirium, drugs and dementia. The clinical syndrome of dementia (changes in two aspects of cognition, including memory, affected functional autonomy or social skills) can be caused by all the conditions listed in Table 9. Some are readily reversible with proper medical treatment. AD is by far the most important cause of dementia (Figure 5).

Delirium, as defined by an acute confusional state, is readily distinguishable from a slowly progressive dementia, but both may co-exist (Table 10). Furthermore, delirium may be a first warning of dementia likely to become apparent within 3 years. Similarly, depression and dementia often co-exist, and there is increasing recognition of depression in the elderly as a potential

- **Depression**
- **Delirium**
- **Drugs**
- **Alzheimer's disease**
- **Non-Alzheimer dementias:**

    Vascular dementias (or multi-infarct dementia)

    Lewy body dementias (or AD with early Parkinson features)

    Frontal lobe dementias (such as Pick's disease)

    Subcortical dementias (such as Parkinson, Huntington or progressive supranuclear palsy)

    Focal cortical atrophy syndromes (such as primary aphasia)

    Metabolic-toxic dementias (such as chronic hypothyroidism or B_{12} deficiency)

    Infections (such as syphilis, neuroAIDS or chronic meningitis)

Table 9
Differential diagnosis of the dementia syndrome.

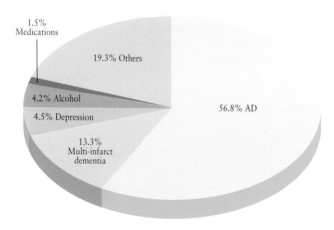

Figure 5
Common causes of dementia (adapted from Katzman and Kawas 1994).

Delirium	Dementia
Abrupt precise onset with identifiable date	Gradual onset that cannot be precisely dated
Acute illness, generally days to weeks, rarely more than 1 month	Chronic illness, characteristically progressing over years
Usually reversible, often completely	Generally irreversible, often chronically progressive
Disorientation early	Disorientation later in the illness, often after months or years
Variability from moment to moment, hour to hour, throughout the day	Much more stable day to day (unless delirium develops)
Prominent physiological changes	Less prominent physiological changes
Clouded, altered, and changing level of consciousness	Consciousness not clouded until terminal
Strikingly short attention span	Attention span not characteristically reduced
Disturbed sleep-wake cycle with hour-to-hour variation	Disturbed sleep-wake cycle with day-night reversal, not hour-to-hour variation
Marked psychomotor changes (hyperactive or hypoactive)	Psychomotor changes characteristically late (unless depression develops)

Table 10
Distinguishing delirium from dementia (see Ham 1997).

early manifestation of AD (Table 11). Patients who have experienced a bout of delirium or depression after age 65 require long-term follow-up for detection of cognitive impairment.

Medical conditions such as hypothyroidism and vitamin B_{12} deficiency may co-exist with AD and are amenable to therapy. All through the course of AD an abrupt deterioration may be caused by a concomitant medical condition (Hogan and McCracken 1999).

Depression	Dementia
Abrupt onset	Insidious onset
Short duration	Long duration
Often previous psychiatric history (including undiagnosed depressive episodes)	No psychiatric history
Highlights disabilities (in particular complains of the memory loss)	Conceals disability (often unaware of memory loss)
"Don't know" answers	"Near-miss" answers
Diurnal variation in mood, but mood generally more consistent	Day-to-day fluctuation in mood
Fluctuating cognitive loss	Stable cognitive loss
Often does not try so hard but is more distressed by losses	Tries hard to perform but is unconcerned
Equal memory loss for recent and remote events	Memory loss greatest for recent events
Depressed mood (if present) occurs first	Memory loss occurs first
Associated with depressed or anxious mood, sleep disturbance, appetite disturbance, and suicidal thoughts	Associated with unsociability, uncooperativeness, hostility, emotional instability, confusion, disorientation, and reduced alertness

Table 11
Distinguishing depression from dementia (see Ham 1997).

All medications in use should be carefully reassessed, particularly those having sedative actions, such as hypnotics and benzodiazepines, or anticholinergic effects, such as over-the-counter cold remedies or anti-tremor Parkinson drugs.

Investigations

Neuropsychological assessment

Detailed neuropsychological assessment may be required in certain early cases of cognitive loss, as there is a grey area between normal aging and AD (Mohr et al 1999). The most sensitive tests of early AD relate to:

- Episodic memory or memory for recent or remote events
- Language, particularly word fluency
- Executive functioning

At the office, the MMSE can be supplemented by asking the patient to draw a clock and set the time at 11:10 (Figure 6). The four criteria that best discriminate between AD patients and controls are:

- Exactly 12 numbers present
- The number 12 at the top
- Two distinguishable hands
- Correct reading of the time

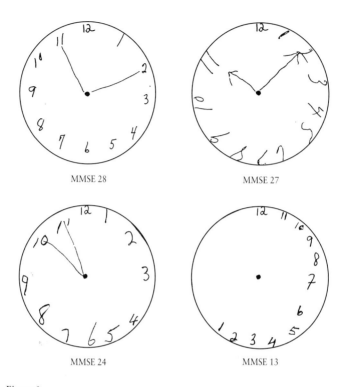

MMSE 28   MMSE 27

MMSE 24   MMSE 13

Figure 6
Illustrations of clock drawings from four Alzheimer patients at different disease stages.

The clock drawing test in combination with a cut-off score of 26/30 on the MMSE was found by Thalmann et al (1996) to have a correct classification rate of 85% (81% sensitivity and 90% specificity) for dementia. Quantitative analysis of the clock drawing is possible in neuropsychological settings, but a qualitative assessment can be readily made by the family practitioner.

Laboratory assessment

A relatively small number of laboratory tests are required in uncomplicated AD (Table 12). HIV testing may be indicated in higher risk groups (Corey-Bloom et al 1995). Brain imaging using computed tomography (CT) or magnetic resonance imaging (MRI) is useful in many (but not all) cases in order to rule out structural brain lesions (tumours, subdural haematomas, hydrocephalus and strokes) (Table 13). These scans essentially document brain atrophy in AD, often asymmetric and involving predominantly the temporal lobes (Figure 7).

- Complete blood count
- Sedimentation rate
- Thyroid function tests
- Serum electrolytes, calcium
- Serum glucose
- Serum BUN/creatine, B_{12}, liver function tests
- Syphilis serology

Table 12
Minimal laboratory work-up for Alzheimer's disease in primary care practice (see CCCAD 1991).

- Age less than 60 years
- Use of anticoagulants or history of bleeding disorder
- Recent head trauma
- History of cancer
- Unexplained neurological symptoms
- Rapid unexplained decline over weeks
- Less than 2 year duration of dementia
- History of urinary incontinence and gait disorders early in the cause of dementia
- New localizing signs
- Gait ataxia

Table 13
Criteria for use of cranial CT in routine clinical practice (see CCCAD 1991).

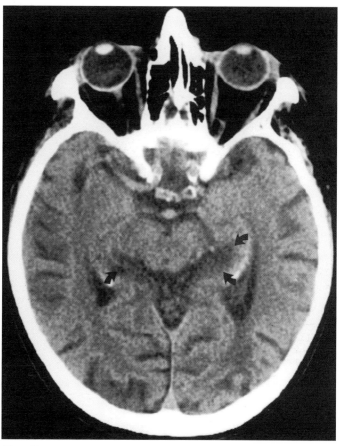

Figure 7
Modified CT axial image of a 72-year-old woman with Alzheimer's disease. Note the moderate dilation of the choroidal–hippocampal fissures (arrows).

Metabolic imaging using positron emission tomography (PET) is used in research settings and may help illustrate drug actions on brain function (Figure 8). The diagnostic value of biological markers such as plasma apoE and CSF tau or other proteins is under investigation, but does not currently replace a reliable history and careful serial clinical assessments (NIA/AAWG 1996).

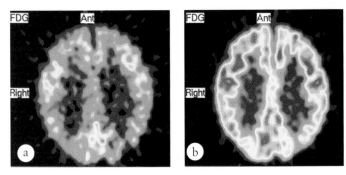

Figure 8
Functional brain imaging of a patient with Alzheimer's disease before (a) and during (b) treatment with a cholinesterase inhibitor. The colour scale indicates regional glucose metabolism after intravenous injection of ^{18}F FDG. A 20–30% increase of regional glucose metabolism can be visualized. With thanks to Dr A Nordberg, Karolinska Institute, Huddinge, Sweden.

Treatment of cognitive deficits

Rationale for treatment

Biopsy and autopsy studies have demonstrated a predominant loss of cholinergic markers in the basal forebrain and neocortex, although other neurotransmitter systems are also altered (Table 14). The reduction in cholinergic markers correlates best with severity of cognitive symptoms as well as pathological markers,

Decreased	Increased
Acetylcholine	Monoamineoxidase B
Serotonine	Galanin
Noradrenaline	
Dopamine	
GABA	
Somatostatin	
Vasopressin	
CRF	
Substance P	
Neuropeptide Y	

Table 14
Neurotransmitter systems altered in Alzheimer's disease (see Feldman and Grundman 1999).

and the best symptomatic therapeutic responses in AD so far have been with pharmacological agents that increase cholinergic activity.

The 'cholinergic hypothesis' has thus driven therapeutic research for AD in the past 20 years, with a variety of drugs targeted to different components of the cholinergic synapse (Table 15 and Figure 9). Other agents, such as propentofylline, act via non-cholinergic mechanisms.

Mode of action	Examples
Precursor loading	choline, lecithin
Neurotransmitter release	besipirdine
Acetylcholinesterase inhibition	tacrine, donepezil, rivastigmine, metrifonate, galanthamine
Muscarinic agonists	milameline, xanomeline, talsaclidine

Table 15
Cholinergic therapy in Alzheimer's disease (see Feldman and Grundman 1999).

Assessment of therapeutic responses

Some of these agents that enhance cholinergic function have demonstrated efficacy in double-blind placebo-controlled conditions, and are or soon will be on the market for general prescription use. However, assessment of the clinical therapeutic response in the primary care setting, where the physician is often alone and has limited time available, is different from the type of assessment that is used in clinical trials. Although complex and lengthy assessments are carried out in randomized trials, even a simple instrument such as the MMSE can show a therapeutic response and is a useful alternative to the

Figure 9
Illustration of cholinergic synaptic activity (a) and sites of action of cholinergic agonists (b).

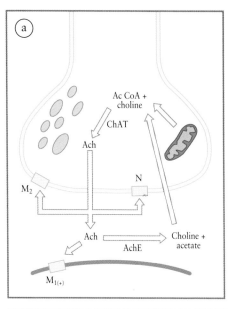

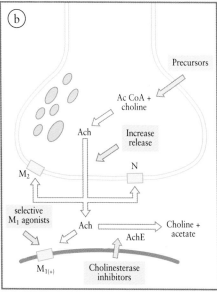

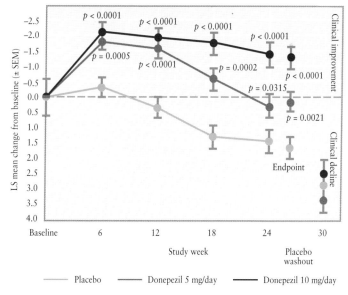

Figure 10
Illustration of therapeutic response to donepezil in an international double-blind, placebo-controlled trial, using the ADAS-cog at regular intervals followed by a 6 week placebo washout period (Gauthier et al 1998).

ADAS-cog, one of the main outcome variables found to be significantly improved in US (Rogers et al 1998) and international (Gauthier et al 1998; Figure 10) studies. The MMSE, in addition to a brief but systematic assessment of function (e.g. ADLs and hobbies), behaviour and moods, based on both carer and patient input, can be used to evaluate therapeutic responsiveness in the primary care setting (Table 16). Evidence from open-label follow-up on donepezil suggests a sustained therapeutic benefit over many years (Figure 11).

- Explain the potential value of Alzheimer-specific drugs and their known side-effects
- Establish the cognitive, functional, behavioural and emotional status before treatment by interviewing the patient and caregiver, and administering MMSE or other structured questionnaire
- Start drug therapy and titrate up following recommendations from the monograph
- Assess efficacy as reflected by improvement in functional abilities (ADL, hobbies, social interaction) and tolerance to treatment at regular intervals
- Add antidepressant if clinically significant depressive symptoms emerge
- Stop treatment if rapid clinical deterioration is observed despite the optimal therapeutic dose or if there are intolerable side-effects
- Continue treatment if there is evidence of functional improvement or slower decline
- Discontinue treatment when the disease has progressed to the severe stage

Table 16
Guidelines for cholinergic drug utilization.

Safety assessment

Cholinergic side-effects (Table 17) should be monitored for dose-adjustment purposes. Fortunately, these side-effects are dose related and show rapid tolerance, particularly for the once daily donepezil (Doody 1999). Laboratory parameters do not need to be serially assessed with certain cholinesterase inhibitors that are chemically unrelated to tacrine (an acridine), which requires serial assessment of liver function tests. Combinations of cholinergic agents are yet to be tested in well structured protocols and should not be attempted in primary care settings for fear of additive cholinergic toxicity. Experience with tacrine and donepezil has shown good compatibility of this cholinesterase inhibitor with commonly used drugs in AD such as antidepressants, neuroleptics and anticonvulsants

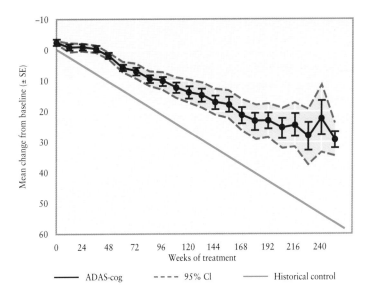

Figure 11
Illustration of sustained therapeutic response to donepezil in open-label follow-up over 4 years, using ADAS-cog, as compared to an historical control group (Friedhoff et al 1998).

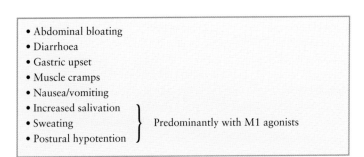

Table 17
Common side-effects of cholinergic agents in Alzheimer's disease.

Non-pharmacological management

The potential value of cognitive rehabilitation or other psychosocial methods as an adjunct to AD specific drug therapy remains to be established but could have a major impact on the size and quality of therapeutic response. Within the next few years we will see an increase in such combination therapies.

Treatment of neuropsychiatric symptoms

Neuropsychiatric symptoms are related to biological changes in AD and include disorders of:

- Mood, usually depression and, rarely, mania
- Perception, with hallucinations and misidentifications
- Thought content with delusions and paranoid ideas
- Behaviour, with aggression, wandering, sexual disinhibition

These features are common, with up to 75% of patients becoming depressed, 33% having persecutory ideas, 20% demonstrating aggressiveness and 15% hallucinations (Figure 11). They cause stress and strain in carers, both at home and in institutions.

Management can be pharmacological and non-pharmacological. Before prescribing a neuroleptic (Table 18), it is important to assess the underlying causes of neuropsychiatric symptoms and to exclude any associated physical illness or distress (such as a distended bladder or colon). Care must be taken in administering neuroleptics because of extrapyramidal side-effects which can be exaggerated in patients with Lewy body dementia. There are few controlled studies establishing the value of one neuroleptic over another, or which symptoms benefit the most. The side-effect profile of a particular drug may be a crucial determinant in whether it is prescribed or not, including parkinsonism, hypotension, sedation, tardive dyskinesias and organ toxicity. Depot preparations may be required in case of low compliance. In addition to neuroleptics, anticonvulsants such as carbamazepine or sodium valproate may be helpful.

Antidepressants (Table 18) are often prescribed in early stages of AD when there is insight on the condition, and in later stages for non-specific agitation. There is little evidence that any particular antidepressant is more effective than another; thus a favourable side-effect profile, and low potential for interaction with other drugs commonly used in elderly patients, will determine the choice of drug. Electroconvulsive therapy (ECT) may be used in extreme circumstances of retardation and withdrawal. Benzodiazepines may be effective sedatives and the risk of dependence is less of a practical problem in older people.

Neuroleptics	Antidepressants
Indications: Agitation, sleeplessness, restlessness (not for simple wandering) **Drugs commonly used:** Haloperidol 0.5 mg QHS to 1.0 mg BID, risperidone 0.5 mg QHS to BID **Side-effects:** Extrapyramidal, decreased cognitive performance	**Selective serotonin uptake inhibitors:** e.g. sertraline 50 mg QD **Atypical antidepressants:** e.g. trazodone 25 to 50 mg QD **Monoamineoxidase inhibitors:** e.g. moclobemide 150 mg BD e.g. selegiline 2.5 to 5 mg QD

Table 18
Pharmacological management of neuropsychiatric disturbances in Alzheimer's disease.

Non-pharmacological therapies include better information for the carers about the nature of neuropsychiatric symptoms, day programs and respite. Reality orientation is generally accepted as being helpful in later stages of AD. Informal individual orientation can be achieved by colour coding areas of the patient's residence and directing them to key areas in the home or ward. Reinforcement of the day and time should be given regularly. Formal reality orientation takes place in small groups and revolves around the provision of repeated stimulation of appropriate orientation. Other approaches under evaluation for AD include validation, reminiscence, music, art or aroma therapy. Behaviour modification can often be the only practical solution for behaviours such as wandering. A close examination of the circumstances surrounding a disruptive behaviour with attention to exacerbating and relieving factors can often result in a clear identification of precipitants, and their removal greatly alleviates the situation.

Patient and family support

AD affects many people besides the patient. The spouse or other primary caregivers will experience a burden increasing in intensity over time; the siblings and children will be concerned about their own genetic risk of developing AD (Maheu and Cohen 1999). A significant loss of income may occur for the primary caregiver, in addition to costs of nursing home care. In countries where the state plays a major role at the later stages of AD through home care support and nursing home placement, a high societal cost is incurred; this is likely to increase dramatically over the next 30 years.

The diagnosis of AD must be carefully documented on serial observations and by questioning reliable informants. Referral for second opinion may be warranted in some cases (Table 19). The primary care physician will often be the one having to reveal the diagnosis and should do so cautiously in individuals suspected of depression. The news may be a relief to some patients and families, since a name will be put to puzzling symptoms. Furthermore, therapeutic options will be increasingly available for effective treatment.

- Continuing uncertainty about diagnosis after initial assessment and follow-up
- Request by family or patient for another opinion
- Presence of significant depression not responding to treatment
- Possible industrial exposure to heavy metals
- Need for help in patient management or support for caregiver
- Need to involve other health professionals in evaluation or management
- Research studies into diagnosis or treatment

Table 19
Criteria for referral to a specialist (from CCCAD 1991).

When the patient and family are ready, a frank discussion about the different stages will help in planning retirement, home care, and institutionalization. The Alzheimer Associations have acquired a large body of experience in educating families about the illness, and offer caregiver support groups. All AD patients and families should be made aware of these lay associations (see Appendix 3).

A novel issue of genetic screening in pre-symptomatic individuals at potentially high risk of AD has emerged. The easily available apoE testing may be requested by family members of a recently diagnosed AD patient. Consensus guidelines on this issue have been published (Table 20). It is currently considered prudent not to perform genetic screening without input from genetic counselling clinics (Figure 12).

- The use of apoE genotyping to predict future risk of AD in symptom-free individuals is not recommended at this time
- In so far as patients with AD are more likely to have an apoE-ε4 allele than are patients with other forms of dementia or individuals without dementia, physicians may choose to use apoE in genotyping as an adjunct to other diagnostic tests for AD
- Since genotyping cannot provide certainty about the presence or absence of AD, it should not be used as the sole diagnostic test
- In deciding whether or not to carry out apoE genotyping for any purpose, physicians and patients should bear in mind that genotype disclosure can have adverse effects on insurability, employability, and the psychosocial status of patients and family members

Table 20
Apolipoprotein E genotyping in Alzheimer's disease (from NIA/AAWG 1996).

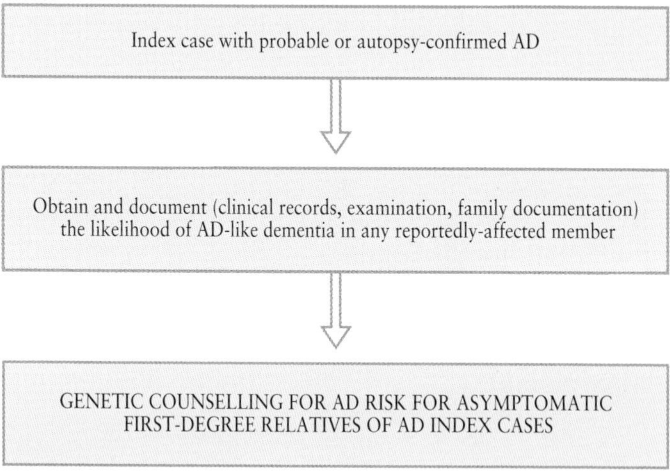

Index case with probable or autopsy-confirmed AD

Obtain and document (clinical records, examination, family documentation) the likelihood of AD-like dementia in any reportedly-affected member

GENETIC COUNSELLING FOR AD RISK FOR ASYMPTOMATIC FIRST-DEGREE RELATIVES OF AD INDEX CASES

Figure 12
Genetic counselling options for Alzheimer's disease (Sadovnick and Lovestone 1999).

The role of the primary care practitioner

Although AD is a common disorder of the elderly (5% of people over age 65), primary care practitioners are aware of only a half of patients under their care, usually at a late stage. Failure of support systems such as the death of a spouse may reveal the AD patient for the first time. The essence of good management of AD is thus one of early diagnosis and proactive care, which should improve the quality of life for patients and carers and lessen the family burden.

Primary care practitioners are well placed to detect AD in the elderly population under his or her care, with a heightened index of suspicion and a systematic approach based on a user-friendly instruments such as the MMSE and drawing of a clock, or any other cognitive assessment tool familiar to him or her. After the appropriate investigations and follow-up visits (Figure 13), once the diagnosis of dementia of the Alzheimer type is made, the practitioner will have to decide how to manage the patient, which includes revealing the diagnosis (Table 21). Sensitivity is needed in this regard, based on the patient's expressed wishes to know his or her diagnosis, and the risk of reactive depression. On the other hand a family member, usually the spouse, needs to know and be well informed about AD. This carer education is facilitated by AD self-help groups.

Early stages	Later stages
• Discuss the diagnosis • Treat concomitant illnesses (particularly depression) • Eliminate non-essential drugs that could interfere with cognition • Advise on will-making and advance directives • Monitor driving ability and safety in use of household appliances • Refer to local AD Association for information and support groups • Discuss referral to genetic counselling services for family members • Discuss use of available AD symptomatic medications • Discuss referral to AD research clinics for experimental therapies	• Help carers find and optimize the preserved functions of the patient • Monitor for and treat neuropsychiatric symptoms • Arrange support through local health services (day programs, respite) • Monitor health and well-being of carers • Plan with carers for smooth transition to nursing home • Make end of life decisions respecting advance directives

Table 21
Responsibilities of primary care practitioners in the management of patients with Alzheimer's disease.

Advice must be given as to the pressing need for advance directives, including designation of a legal guardian for future needs, through a lawyer or notary (Peisah and Brodaty 1994). Driving is also a medico-legal responsibility that requires monitoring on the part of the practitioner with the help of the carer and sometimes the professional assessment of an occupational therapist (Hunt et al 1993). Fortunately few countries or states require the immediate notification of the diagnosis of AD to the motor vehicle bureaus, but all require a careful follow-up of driving abilities as the disease evolves over time. Driving restrictions to familiar areas, usually with a navigator, are a useful compromise, until cognitive loss or neuropsychiatric manifestations require cessation of driving altogether. The practitioner will also be asked about the patient's competence to make a will and manage his or her finances. Since there is no international gold standard as to the determination of competence, carefully documented notes in the medical chart, including serial MMSE or other test scores, will be extremely useful.

Most practitioners care for AD patients in the community setting, and it is essential to alleviate the burden of caring by family members as much as possible. This can be achieved by advice about home environment and arranging support through local health services, which may include social service, nursing and occupational therapy assessment. Day programs and respite care are available in most areas, often delaying transfer to institutional settings (Mittelman et al 1996). The latter will eventually be required, with appropriate assistance from the practitioner and the primary care team (Downs 1996).

Future prospects

Primary care physicians already look after most patients with AD, either in the community or in long-term institutions.

An office evaluation for dementia is not recommended for all aged individuals but rather when certain symptoms are found (Table 22). This will require more than one short visit (Figure 13).

- Memory or other cognitive complaints with or without functional impairment
- Elderly patients with questionable competency
- Depressed or anxious patients with cognitive complaints
- Suspicion of cognitive impairment on routine interview

Table 22
Individuals in need of assessment for dementia (from the Report of the Quality Standards Subcommittee of the AAN 1994).

The availability of new therapeutic agents will be an incentive for earlier diagnosis and more frequent assessments. Research on the value of such agents in the moderate to severe stages of AD is underway, particularly in the area of delaying emergence of behavioural symptoms, or controlling existing symptoms

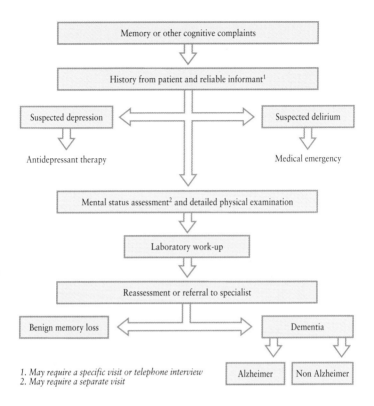

Figure 13
Algorithm for the diagnosis of dementia in primary care practice.

without the side-effects of neuroleptics. Sensitive ethical issues must be considered in these stages, when the patient is not competent to give full informed consent, but should not be denied potentially effective therapy.

Current agents are primarily symptomatic, but a number of aetiological hypothesis are leading to a stabilization approach. The knowledge gained on protective and risk factors for AD in combination with stabilization agents could lead to a truly preventive approach to AD in the next few years.

Appendix 1:
User-friendly Mini-Mental State Examination

What is the day of the week?	__ /1
What is the month?	__ /1
What is the date?	__ /1
What is the season?	__ /1
What is the year?	__ /1
What city are we in?	__ /1
What is the county (or state or province)?	__ /1
What is the country?	__ /1
What is the name of the hospital (or building)?	__ /1
What floor are we on?	__ /1
Repeat till you remember: ball, car, man (score after 2 trials)	__ /3
Spell the word "WORLD"; now try to spell it backwards DLROW	__ /5
What were the three words that you were asked to remember?	__ /3
What is this called? (Show a watch)	__ /1

Cont'd.

What is this called? (Show a pencil)	__ /1
Repeat after me "No ifs ands or buts")	__ /1
Read and do what is written down: CLOSE YOUR EYES	__ /1
Write a short sentence	__ /1
Copy this drawing (2 interlocking pentagons)	__ /1
Take this paper in your left (or right if left handed) hand	__ /1
fold it in half and	__ /1
put it on the floor	__ /1
TOTAL SCORE	___ /30

Modified from Folstein et al 1975.

Appendix 2:
Diagnostic criteria

Diagnostic criteria of dementia of the Alzheimer type

Development of multiple cognitive deficits manifested by both:

1. Memory impairment (impaired ability to learn new information or to recall previously learned information)

2. One or more of:
   — aphasia
   — apraxia
   — agnosia
   — disturbance in executive functioning

These cognitive deficits cause a significant impairment in social or occupational functioning and represent a significant decline from a previous level of functioning.

Gradual onset and continuing cognitive decline.

Cognitive deficits that are not due to:

1. Other CNS conditions that cause progressive deficits in memory and cognition (e.g. cerebrovascular disease, Parkinson's, Huntington's, subdural haematoma, normal-pressure hydrocephalus, brain tumour)

2. Systemic conditions that are known to cause dementia (e.g. hypothyroidism, vitamin B_{12} or folic acid deficiency, niacin deficiency, hypercalcaemia, neurosyphilis, HIV infection)

3. Substance-induced condition (e.g. alcohol, sedatives)

Cont'd.

The cognitive deficits do not occur exclusively during the course of a delirium.

Disturbance that is not better accounted for by another primary psychiatric disorder such as major depression or schizophrenia.

Modified from DSM-IV (APA 1994).

Diagnostic criteria of delirium

- Disturbances of consciousness with change in cognition that is not better accounted for by a dementia
- Develops over hours to days
- Fluctuates during the course of the day
- Impaired ability to focus, sustain or shift attention
- Impaired cognition (memory, orientation, language) or perceptual disturbance (misinterpretation, illusions, hallucinations)
- Associated with sleep-wake cycle, psychomotor, emotional or EEG disturbance
- Evidence that the disturbance is caused by a general medical condition, substance intoxication or withdrawal, or multiple aetiologies

Modified from DSM-IV (APA 1994).

Diagnostic criteria for dementia with Lewy bodies (DLB)

Progressive cognitive decline interfering with social or occupational functioning; memory loss may not be an early feature.

One (possible DLB) or two (probable DLB) of:

1. Fluctuating cognition with pronounced variations in attention and alertness
2. Recurrent visual hallucinations
3. Spontaneous motor features of Parkinsonism

Modified from McKeith et al 1996.

Diagnostic criteria for frontotemporal dementia

Behavioural disorder:
- Insidious onset and slow progression
- Early loss of personal and social awareness
- Early signs of disinhibition
- Mental rigidity and inflexibility
- Hyperorality, stereotyped and perseverative behaviours

Affective symptoms:
- Depression, anxiety
- Somatic preoccupations
- Emotional unconcern, amimia

Cont'd.

Speech disorder:
- Reduction and stereotypy of speech
- Echolalia and perseveration

Physical signs:
- Early primitive reflexes and incontinence
- Late akinesia, rigidity, tremor

Modified from The Lund Manchester Groups 1994.

Diagnostic criteria for vascular dementia

- Presence of a dementia syndrome
- Focal neurological signs and symptoms or neuroimaging evidence of cerebrovascular disease judged aetiologically related to the disturbance
- Symptoms not occurring exclusively during the course of a delirium

Modified from DSM-IV (APA 1994).

Appendix 3:
Alzheimer's Disease International contact information

Head office
Alzheimer's Disease International
45–46 Lower Marsh
London SE1 7RG
United Kingdom
Tel: +44 171 620 3011
Fax: +44 171 401 7351
E-mail: adi@alzdisint.demon.co.uk
Web: www.alzdisint.demon.co.uk
Executive Director: Elizabeth Rimmer

Full members

Argentina
ALMA (Asociación de Lucha contra el Mal de Alzheimer)
Lacarra No. 78
1407 Capital Federal
Buenos Aires
Argentina
Tel/fax: +54 1 671 1187
E-mail: alma@satlink.com.ar

Australia
Alzheimer's Association Australia
PO Box 42
North Ryde
NSW 2113
Australia
Tel: +61 2 98050100
Fax: +61 2 98051665
E-mail: admin@alznsw.asn.au
Web: www.alznsw.asn.au

Austria
Alzheimer Angehorige Austria
Obere Augartenstrasse 26–28
1020 Vienna
Austria
Tel: +43 1 332 5166
Fax: +43 1 334 2141
E-mail: alzheimeraustria@via.at

Belgium
Ligue Alzheimer
Clinique le peri
4B rue Montagne Ste Walburge
4000 Liège
Belgium
Tel: +32 4 225 8793
Fax: +32 4 226 7231

Brazil
FEBRAZ Federação Brasileira de Associações de Alzheimer
Av Paulista, 726-cj 501
São Paulo
SP Brasil 01310-100
Tel/fax: +55 11 288 7428
E-mail: abrz@wm.com.br
Web: www.wm.com.br/alzheimer

Canada
Alzheimer Society of Canada
20 Eglinton Ave W
Suite 1200
Toronto
Ontario M4R 1K8
Canada
Tel: +1 416 488 8772
Fax: +1 416 488 3778
E-mail: info@alzheimer.ca
Web: www.alzheimer.ca

Chile
Corporación Chilena de la Enfermedad de Alzheimer y Afecciones
    Similares
General Parra 674
Providencia
Santiago
Chile
Tel: +56 2 236 0846
Fax: +56 2 235 6815/222 5515

Colombia
Asociación Colombiana de Alzheimer y Desórdenes Relacionados
Calle 69 A No 10–16
Santa Fe de Bogota DC
Colombia
Tel: +57 1 248 1614
Fax: +57 1 321 7691

Denmark
Alzheimerforeningen
Sankt Lukas vej 13
2900 Hellerup
Denmark
Tel: +45 39 40 04 88
Fax: +45 39 61 66 69

Finland
Alzheimer Society of Finland
Luotsikatu 4E
00160 Helsinki
Finland
Tel: +358 9 6226 2013
Fax: +358 9 6226 2020
E-mail: tarja.tapaninen@alzheimer.fi
Web: www.alzheimer.fi

France
Association France Alzheimer
21 boulevard Montmartre
75002 Paris
France
Tel: +33 1 4297 5241
Fax: +33 1 4296 0470
Web: www.infobiogen.fr

Germany
Deutsche Alzheimer Gesellschaft
Kanstrasse 152
10623 Berlin
Germany
Tel: +49 30 315 057 33
Fax: +49 30 315 057 35
E-mail: deutsche.alzheimer.ges@t.online.de

Greece
Greek Society of Alzheimer's Disease and Related Disorders
92 Egnatia Street
546 23 Thessaloniki
Hellas/Greece 56625
Tel/fax: +30 31 264 380
E-mail: evita@psy.auth.gr

Guatemala
Asociación Grupo Ermita
10a Calle 11–63
Zona 1, Apartamento B
PO Box 2978
01901 Guatemala
Tel/fax: +502 2 381122

Hong Kong
Hong Kong Alzheimer's Disease and Brain Failure Association
c/o GF Wang Lai House
Wang Tau Hom Estate
Kowloon
Hong Kong
Tel: +852 279 43010
Fax: +852 233 84820

India
Alzheimer's and Related Disorders Society of India
Guruvayoor Road
PO Arthat
Kunnamkulam 680 503
Kerala
India
Tel: +91 488 522 415
Fax: +91 488 522 347
E-mail: alzheimr@ind2.vsnl.net.in
Web: www.alzheimr.com

Ireland
Alzheimer's Society of Ireland
Alzheimer's House
40 Northumberland Avenue
Dunlaoghaire, Co. Dublin
Ireland
Tel: +353 1 284 6616
Fax: +353 1 284 6030
E-mail: alzheim@iol.ie

Israel
Alzheimer's Association of Israel
PO Box 8261
Ramat Gan
Israel 52181
Tel: +972 3 578 7660
Fax: +972 3 578 7661
E-mail: aai@netvision.net.il
Web: www2.netvision.net.il/~aai/

Italy

Federazione Alzheimer Italia
Via Marino 7
20121 Milano
Italy
Tel: +39 2 80 9767
Fax: +39 2 87 5781
E-mail: alzit@tin.it
Web: www.alzheimer.it

Japan

Association of Family Caring for Demented Elderly
c/o Kyoto Social Welfare Hall
Horikawa-Marutamachi
Kamigyo-Ku, Kyoto
Japan 602
Tel: +81 75 811 8195
Fax: +81 75 811 8188
E-mail: afcdejpn@mbox.kyoto-inet.or.jp
Web: www2f.meshnet.or.jp/~boke/boke2.htm

Korea

Association of Family Caring for Demented Elderly in Korea
#52, Machon 2-Dong
Songpa-Ku
Seoul 138–122
Korea
Tel: +82 2 431 9963
Fax: +82 2 203 9421
E-mail: AFCDE97@decom.chollian.co.kr

Luxembourg

Association Luxembourg Alzheimer
45 rue Nicolas Hein
Luxembourg BP 5021
L-1050 Luxembourg
Tel: +352 4 21676
Fax: +352 4 21679
E-mail: ala@selection.line.net
Web: www.alzheimer-europe.org/luxembourg

Mexico

AMAES
Insurgentes Sur No. 594–402
Col. Del Valle, Mexico 12
DF 03100 Mexico
Tel/fax: +525 523 1526
E-mail: amaes@data.net.mx

Netherlands
Alzheimerstichting
Post Bus 183
3980 CD Bunnik
The Netherlands
Tel: +31 30 659 6285
Fax: +31 30 659 6283
E-mail: info@alzheimer-ned.nl
Web: www.alzheimer-ned.nl

New Zealand
Alzheimer's Society NZ
Box 2808
Christchurch
New Zealand
Tel: +64 3 365 1590
Fax: +64 3 379 8744
E-mail: alzheimers@alzheimers.org.nz

Poland
Polish Alzheimer's Association
000-682 Warszawa
ul.Hoza 54/1
Poland
Tel/fax: +48 22 622 11 22

Puerto Rico
Asociación de Alzheimer de Puerto Rico
Apartado 362026
San Juan
Puerto Rico 00936-2026
Tel: +1 787 727 4151
Fax: +1 787 727 4890
E-mail: aadrpr@caribe.net

Romania
Romanian Alzheimer Society
Bd. Mihail Kogalniceanu nr 95A
Sc. A, Et 1, Ap. 8 Sector 5
Bucharest
Romania 70603
Tel: +40 1 686 3470
Tel/fax: +40 1 311 3471
E-mail: alzsocro@px.ro
Web: www.alzheimer-europe.org/romania

Scotland

Alzheimer Scotland — Action on Dementia
22 Drumsheugh Gardens
Edinburgh EH3 7RN
Scotland
Tel: +44 131 243 1453
Fax: +44 131 243 1450
E-mail: alzheimer@alzscot.org

Singapore

Alzheimer's Disease Association
Blk 151 Toa Payoh Lor 2 #01-468
Singapore 1231
Tel: +65 353 8734
Fax: +65 353 8518
E-mail: alzheimers.tp@pacific.net.sg

South Africa

Alzheimer's and Related Disorders Association
PO Box 81183
Parkhurst
Johannesburg 2120
South Africa
Tel: +27 11 478 2234/5/6
Fax: +27 11 478 2251
E-mail: alzheimerssa@icon.co.za

Spain

Federated Association of Family Alzheimer Associations
Pintor Maeztu, 2-Bajo
31008 Pamplona
Spain
Tel/fax: +34 48 260 304
E-mail: alzheimer@cin.es

Sweden

Alzheimer's Society of Sweden
Sunnanväg 14S
222 26 Lund
Sweden
Tel: +46 46 14 73 18
Fax: +46 46 18 89 76
E-mail: alzheimf@algonet.se
Web: www.psykiatr.lu.se/alzheimer/

Switzerland
Association Alzheimer's Suisse
Rue Pestalozzi 16
CH-1400 Yverdon-les-Bains
Switzerland
Tel: +41 24 426 2000
Fax: +41 24 426 2167
E-mail: alz@bluewin.ch

United Kingdom
Alzheimer's Disease Society
Gordon House
10 Greencoat Place
London SW1P 1PH
United Kingdom
Tel: +44 171 306 0606
Fax: +44 171 306 0808
E-mail: info@alzheimers.org.uk
Web: www.alzheimers.org.uk

United States
Alzheimer's Association
919 N Michigan Avenue
Suite 1000
Chicago, Illinois 60611
USA
Tel: +1 312 335 8700
Fax: +1 312 335 1110
E-mail: info@alz.org
Web: www.alz.org

Uruguay
Asociación Uruguaya de Alzheimer y Similares
Casilla de Correo 18951
Montevideo
Uruguay
Tel: +598 2 40 87 97
E-mail: audasur@adinet.com.uy

Venezuela
Fundación Alzheimer de Venezuela
Apartado Postal No. 113
Carmelitas 1010, Reg. Postal 01
Caracas
Venezuela 1010
Tel/fax : +582 62 94 95
E-mail: alzven@cantv.net

Provisional members

Cuba
Centro Iberoamericano de la Tercera Edad
Hospital Universitario 'Calixto Garcia'
Calle G y 27 Vedado
Ciudad Habana
Tel: +537 33 3864
Fax: +537 33 3319

Czech Republic
Ceska Alzheimerovska Spolecnost
Simunkova 1600
Prague 8
Czech Republic 18200
Tel: +4202 88 36 76
Fax: +4202 71019 335
E-mail: Gerontocentrum@telecom.cz

Dominican Republic
Asociación Dominicana de Alzheimer y Trastornos Relacionados
Apartado Postal #3321
Santo Domingo
Republica Dominicana
Tel: +1 809 221 6115
Fax: +1 809 562 4690
E-mail: dr.pedro@codetel.net.do

Ecuador
Alzheimer's Disease Ecuador
Avenida de la Prensa #5204 y Avenida del Maestro
Quito
Ecuador
Tel/fax: +593 2 595 767/594 997

Turkey
Alzheimer Association
Cakiraga Cami Sok Kafkas,is Hani
29/11 Aksaray
Istanbul
Turkey
Tel: +90 212 588 2108
Fax: +90 212 588 2254

Bibliography

Allen NHP, Burns A. The noncognitive features of dementia. *Reviews in Clinical Gerontology* 1995; **5**:57–75.

American Psychiatric Association. *Diagnostic and Statistical Manual of Mental Disorders*, 4th edn. APA: Washington DC, 1994.

Bouchard RW, Rossor MN. Typical clinical features. In: Gauthier S, ed. *Clinical Diagnosis and Management of Alzheimer's Disease*, 2nd edn. Martin Dunitz: London, 1999:57–71.

Canadian Study of Health and Aging. Study methods and prevalence of dementia in Canada. *Canadian Medical Association Journal* 1994a; **150**:899–913.

Canadian Study of Health and Aging. Risk factors for Alzheimer's disease in Canada. *Neurology* 1994b; **44**:2073–2080.

Carrier L, Brodaty H. Mood and behaviour management. In: Gauthier S, ed. *Clinical Diagnosis and Management of Alzheimer's Disease*, 2nd edn. Martin Dunitz: London, 1999:229–248.

Corey-Bloom J, Thal LJ, Galasko D et al. Diagnosis and evaluation of dementia. *Neurology* 1995; **45**:211–218.

Doody RS. Clinical profile of donepezil in the treatment of Alzheimer's disease. *Gerontology* 1999; **45 (Suppl. 1)**:23–32.

Downs MG. The role of general practice and the primary care team in dementia diagnosis and management. *International Journal of Geriatric Psychiatry* 1996; **11**:937–942.

Evans DA, Funkenstein H, Albert MS et al. Prevalence of Alzheimer's disease in a community population of older persons; higher than previously reported. *Journal of the American Medical Association* 1989; **262**:2551–2556.

Feldman H, Grundman M. Symptomatic treatments for Alzheimer's disease. In: Gauthier S, ed. *Clinical Diagnosis and Management of Alzheimer's Disease*, 2nd edn. Martin Dunitz: London, 1999:249–268.

Folstein MF, Folstein SE, McHugh PR. Mini Mental State: a practical method for grading the cognitive state of patients for the clinician. *Journal of Psychiatric Research* 1975; **12**:189–198.

Fontaine S, Bourgouin P. Structural brain imaging in Alzheimer's disease. In: Gauthier S, ed. *Clinical Diagnosis and Management of Alzheimer's Disease*, 2nd edn. Martin Dunitz: London, 1999:107–116.

Friedhoff LT, Ieni JR, Rogers SL, Pratt RD. Donepezil provides long-term clinical benefits for patients with Alzheimer's disease. *Presented at the 21st Collegium Internationale Neuropsychopharmacologicum Congress (CINP), Glasgow, 12–16 July 1998.*

Gauthier S, Rossor M, Hecker J et al. Results from a multinational phase III clinical trial of donepezil in Alzheimer's disease. *Presented at the 5th International Geneva/Springfield Alzheimer Symposium, Geneva, 15–18 April 1998.*

Gauthier S, Thal L, Rossor M. The future diagnosis and management of Alzheimer's disease. In: Gauthier S, ed. *Clinical Diagnosis and Management of Alzheimer's Disease*, 2nd edn. Martin Dunitz: London, 1999:369–378.

Geldmacher DS, Whitehouse PJ. Evaluation of dementia. *New England Journal of Medicine* 1996; **335**:330–336.

Gélinas I, Auer S. Functional autonomy. In: Gauthier S, ed. *Clinical Diagnosis and Management of Alzheimer's Disease*, 2nd edn. Martin Dunitz: London, 1999:213–226.

Ham RJ. Confusion, dementia and delirium. In: Ham RJ, Sloane PD, eds. *Primary Care Geriatrics, A Case Based Approach*, 3rd edn. Mosby: St-Louis, 1997:217–259.

Hogan DB, McCracken PN. Associated medical conditions and complications. In: Gauthier S, ed. *Clinical Diagnosis and Management of Alzheimer's Disease*, 2nd edn. Martin Dunitz: London, 1999:279–291.

Hunt L, Marris JC, Edwards E, Wilson BS. Driving performance in persons with mild senile dementia of the Alzheimer type. *Journal of the American Geriatric Society* 1993; **41**:747–753.

Hux MJ, O'Brien BJ, Iskedjian M et al. Relation between severity of Alzheimer's disease and costs of caring. *Canadian Medical Association Journal* 1998; **159**:457–465.

Katzman R, Kawas C. The epidemiology of dementia and Alzheimer's disease. In: Terry RD, Katzman R, Bick KL (eds) *Alzheimer's Disease*. Raven Press: New York, 1994:105–122.

Levy R. Cholinergic treatment of Alzheimer's disease. In: Burns A, Levy R, eds. *Dementia*. Chapman & Hall: London, 1994:511–518.

The Lund Manchester Groups. Clinical and neuropathological criteria for frontotemporal dementia. *Journal of Neurology, Neurosurgery and Psychiatry* 1994; **57**:416–418.

Maheu S, Cohen CA. Support of families. In: Gauthier S, ed. *Clinical Diagnosis and Management of Alzheimer's Disease*, 2nd edn. Martin Dunitz: London, 1999:307–318.

McKeith IG, Galasko D, Kosaka K et al. Consensus guidelines for the clinical and pathological diagnosis of dementia with Lewy bodies (DLB): report of the consortium on DLB international workshop. *Neurology* 1996; **47**:1113–1124.

McKhann G, Drachman D, Folstein M et al. Clinical diagnosis of Alzheimer's disease: report of the NINCDS-ADRDA workgroup. *Neurology* 1984; **34**:939–944.

Mittelman MS, Ferris SH, Shulman E et al. A family intervention to delay nursing home placement of patients with Alzheimer's disease. *Journal of the American Medical Association* 1996; **276**:1725–1731.

Mohr E, Dastoor D, Claus JJ. Neuropsychological assessment. In: Gauthier S, ed. *Clinical Diagnosis and Management of Alzheimer's Disease*, 2nd edn. Martin Dunitz: London, 1999:93–106.

National Institute on Aging/Alzheimer's Association Working Group. Apolipoprotein E genotyping in Alzheimer's disease. *Lancet* 1996; **347**:1091–1095.

Organizing Committee, Canadian Consensus Conference on the Assessment of Dementia. *Canadian Medical Association Journal* 1991; **144**:851–853.

Peisah C, Brodaty H. Dementia and the will-making process. *Medical Journal of Australia* 1994; **161**:381–384.

Poirier J, Danik M, Blass JP. Pathophysiology of the Alzheimer syndrome. In: Gauthier S, ed. *Clinical Diagnosis and Management of Alzheimer's Disease*, 2nd edn. Martin Dunitz: London, 1999:17–32.

Poirier J, Davignon J, Bouthillier D et al. Apolipoprotein E polymorphism and Alzheimer's disease. *Lancet* 1993; **342**:697–699.

Reisberg B. Alzheimer's disease. In: Sadavoy J, Lazarus LW, Jarvik LF, Grossberg GT, eds. *Comprehensive Review of Geriatric Psychiatry - II*, 2nd edn. American Association for Geriatric Psychiatry, American Psychiatric Press Inc: Washington DC, 1996:401–458.

Reisberg B, Ferris SH, DeLeon MJ et al. The global deterioration scale for assessment of primary degenerative dementia. *American Journal of Psychiatry* 1982; **139**:1136–1139.

Report of the Quality Standards Subcommittee of the American Academy of Neurology. Practice parameters for diagnosis and evaluation of dementia. *Neurology* 1994; **44**:2203–2206.

Rogers SL, Farlow MR, Doody RS et al, and the Donepezil Study Group. A 24-week double-blind, placebo-controlled trial of donepezil in patients with Alzheimer's disease. *Neurology* 1998; **50**:136–145.

Rossor MN. Management of neurological disorders: dementia. *Journal of Neurology, Neurosurgery and Psychiatry* 1994; **57**:1451–1456.

Sadovnick AD, Lovestone S. Genetic counselling. In: Gauthier S, ed. *Clinical Diagnosis and Management of Alzheimer's Disease,* 2nd edn. Martin Dunitz: London, 1999:355–365.

Terry RD, Masliah E, Hansen LA. Structural basis of the cognitive alterations in Alzheimer's disease. In: Terry RD, Katzman R, Bick KL, eds. *Alzheimer Disease.* Raven Press: New York, 1994:179–196.

Thalman B, Mansch AU, Ermini-Fiinfschilling D et al. Improved screening for dementia: combining the Clock Drawing Test and the Mini-Mental Status Examination. *Presented at the 4th International Nice/Springfield Alzheimer Symposium, Nice, 10–14 April 1996.*

Index

Page numbers in *italic* refer to the illustrations